THE COMPLETE GUIDE TO INTERMITTENT FASTING

The Complete Guide To Detox The Body, Reset Metabolism, Lose Weight, And Delay Aging

Audrey Davidson

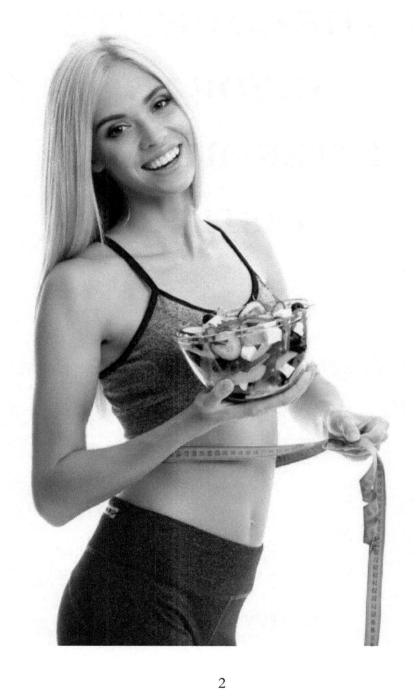

Table of Contents

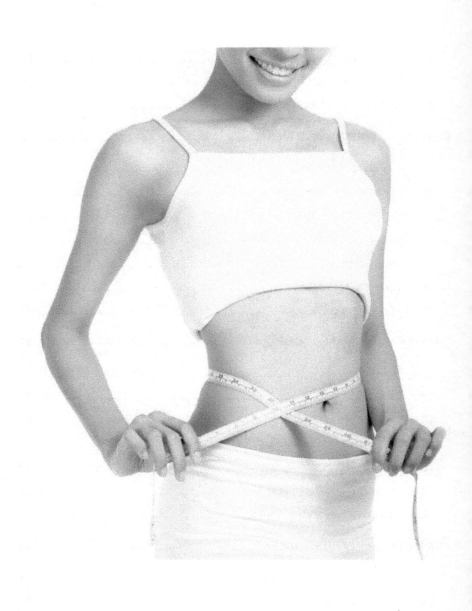

Introduction

Intermittent fasting for women over 50 may help reduce breast cancer risk, according to a study published in the journal Cancer Research.

Intermittent fasting is becoming more popular as the years go on. While most people are familiar with this for men, women over 50 can benefit from it too.

This kind of fasting is a dieting technique that involves short periods of fasting every day.

Intermittent fasting is a diet that allows you to eat all the food you want during a specific fasting window. It can help you lose weight. However, this kind of fasting is more than just losing weight.

Intermittent fasting for women over 50 is all about eating fewer Calories while still nourishing your body. During the fasting period, you'll eat 500 calories on non-fasting days and 1,000 Calories on fasting days.

Intermittent fasting is when you restrict calories or eating hours during the week. It is the opposite of what we usually do, which is to eat a certain amount every day of the week (a diet). This is frequently referred to as "caloric restriction" and it has been shown to prolong life in many research studies.

When you restrict your calories such as when you fast, your body is forced to use more of its own fat for energy. This is not captured by most people because they are in a calorie deficit and thus not eating enough to give their bodies the energy needed. The caloric restriction is part of intermittent fasting as opposed to dieting where calorie restriction is only one part of the equation.

There are a number of different ways to do intermittent fasting, the most common one being eating within 8 hours and fasting the rest of the time. The less common way is called "time-restricted feeding" because you are only allowed to eat during a specific time window. This can be done as a specific eating window every day such as 12-8 pm or 6-10 pm. Most people will be doing this on a weekly basis by either restricting breakfast or dinner (or both) on the day before their weekly fast.

Fasting intermittently is one of the best methods people have for reducing excess weight off but holding healthy weight on, and it needs relatively least behavior modification. This is a positive idea because it ensures intermittent fasting fits under the easy enough task that one will simply do it, however significant enough that it can make a transformation. Intermittent fasting shifts hormone levels to promote weight reduction.

In addition to reducing insulin in the bloodstream and increasing growth hormone levels, it enhances the production of the burning fat hormone known as noradrenaline or norepinephrine.

Studies suggest that a very effective method for weight reduction may be intermittent fasting. Short-term fasting can raise the body's metabolic rate by 3.6 to 14 percent due to these hormones' changes. By encouraging one to eat less, burn additional calories, by manipulating all calorie calculation aspects, intermittent fasting induces weight loss.

Intermittent fasting (IF) can sound very restrictive, but there are many strategies and plans out there to help you make it easier to do. For example, you can switch from eating breakfast every day to fasting breakfast every day or you can just start by skipping dinner on a specific day each week.

Chapter 1. What Is Intermittent Fasting?

During intermittent fasting, you would not be pressured to deprive yourself throughout the day, also mentioned as IF. It also doesn't grant you a license during the period of non-fasting to eat loads of unhealthy food. You consume within a fixed window of time, instead of consuming meals and treats all day. Intermittent fasting is an eating pattern model that requires daily, short-term fasts or limited or no food intake at times.

Most individuals know intermittent fasting as losing weight assistance. Intermittent fasting is a lifestyle that allows people to consume fewer calories, leading to weight loss over time.

Without being on an insane diet or consuming the calories to nil, it's a perfect way to get healthy. Most of the time, when one begins intermittent fasting, they'll aim to maintain their calories the same as during a shortened time; most people consume larger meals. In comparison, prolonged fasting is a healthy way to preserve body mass while becoming lean. But most notably, intermittent fasting is among the most beneficial way to be in shape with many other benefits. This is an easy way to get the desired results. If performed properly, intermittent fasting will have valuable advantages, like weight reduction, type 2 diabetes reversal, and several other aspects. Plus, this will save time and resources for you.

Intermittent fasting is successful because it makes it possible for the amount of insulin and blood sugar to reach a low level. The body's fat-storing enzyme is insulin. Fat moves into the fat cells and gets absorbed when insulin levels are high in the blood; if insulin level is low, Fat will move and burn out of Fat cells. In short, IF is when food is readily available, but you prefer not to consume it. This may be over any period of time, from several hours to a couple of days, or sometimes a week or more under strict medical monitoring. You can begin fasting at any moment of your choice, and you can end a fast at your will, too.

You fast intermittently if you don't consume food by choice. For instance, between dinner and breakfast, till the following day, you will not eat and fast for around 12 to 14 hours. Intermittent fasting can, in that way, be deemed a part of daily life.

The Science Behind It

Like any idea of eating that quickly takes over health and diet cultures, intermittent fasting has been suspected to be a fad. Still, the evidence behind fasting's advantages is already clear— and increasing.

There are several hypotheses as to why intermittent fasting performs so well, but tension has to do with the most widely studied — and most proven gain.

The term stress has been vilified continuously, but the body profits from some stress. Exercise, for example, is technically stress on the body (especially on the muscles and the cardiovascular system). Still, this specific stress ultimately makes the body better as long as you implement the correct amount of recovery period into your exercise plan.

Intermittent fasting stresses the body in the same way that exercise does; it brings the cells under moderate tension as you refuse the body food for a certain period. Cells respond to this tension over time by studying how to better cope with it. It has an improved ability to resist illness because the body becomes better at dealing with pain.

All About Intermittent Fasting

Over the age of 50, it is increasingly difficult for a woman to lose weight, and we are obsessed with those extra pounds that accumulate in areas where we do not want them to, such as hips and love handles. Intermittent fasting is an alternative to the usual diets. It can also become a way of life if you think of the countless benefits that calorie restriction brings to the body and mind.

The different intermittent fasting types allow us to evaluate and choose the most suitable one for us, adapting it to our needs and lifestyle.

It is necessary to maintain a balanced and healthy diet, rich in vegetables and whole grains, and that provides all the macronutrients needed by the body and the right amount of Fat (preferably vegetable) and avoid junk food seasoned and too salty. All in all, however, you can eat anything, even taking a few whims from time to time.

Fasting has positive implications for the health of women over 50. Science has shown that reducing calorie intake prolongs life because it acts on the metabolic function of longevity genes, reduces senile diseases, cancer, cardiovascular diseases, and neurodegenerative ones such as Alzheimer's and Parkinson's disease. Also, especially for women over 50, it has multiple benefits on mood, fights depression, and contributes to energy, libido, and concentration. And as if that weren't enough, it gives the skin a better look.

To start this type of "diet," you must first be in good health, and in any case, before starting, it is always better to consult your doctor. The female body is susceptible to calorie restriction because the hypothalamus, a gland in the brain responsible for hormone production, is stimulated. These hormones risk going haywire with a drastic reduction in Calories or too long a fast. Therefore, the advice is to start gradually, perhaps introducing some vegetable snacks during fasting hours (fennel, lettuce, endive, and radicchio).

As mentioned, in women, intermittent fasting works differently than in men. Sometimes it is more difficult for women to get results. Physiological and weight benefits are still possible but sometimes require a different approach. Also, intermittent fasting on non-consecutive days is better able to keep those annoying hormones under control. Various scientific evidence shows that to achieve Fat loss, fasting must be tailored to the sex.

For women, in particular, there are specific biological truths about fasting that will prevent you from achieving your goals of a better body and fitness if you ignore them. But there may be variations that allow you to overcome these problems. Fasting can prove to be a convenient and effective way to optimize your health and make you feel better, but only if it is done in a certain way: the best for each of us.

Fasting, after all, represents the easiest and, at the same time, powerful detoxification and regeneration therapy that we can offer to cells and the whole organism. Putting certain functions at physiological rest does not mean that organs and tissues go on stand-by. On the contrary, thanks to the absence of a continuous metabolic commitment, they can dedicate themselves to something else, activating all those processes of self-repair, catabolism, excretion, and cell turnover that only in the absence of nutrients can take place at the highest levels.

Chapter 2. The Best Intermittent Fasting Types to Follow

5.2 Fasting

The 5:2 eating routine is another reasonable alternative. This fast encourages you to ordinarily eat for five days during the week and fast for the other two days and only eat about 600 Calories. This is at times called the Easy Diet, as well. It's suggested that on these fasting days, individuals will eat around 500 to 600 Calories.

You'll ordinarily eat all week long, for instance, and on Monday and Thursdays, you'll have just two little dinners within about 500 Calories. You can pick anytime as your fasting days, as long as you don't have them in consecutive order. Pick your two busiest days of the week. What's more, make them your fasting days.

There aren't numerous reports out there about the 5:2 eating regimen, yet it will give the greater part of the advantages you're finding with intermittent fasting. You can do it without the need to think the entire day about making dinners.

16/8 Fasting

16/8 intermittent fasting includes restricting the utilization of food sources and calorie-containing drinks to a set window of eight hours out of each day and avoiding nourishment for the remaining 16 hours. It can be repeated often — from only a single time or two times a week to consistently, contingent upon your preference. 16/8 intermittent fasting has soared in popularity as of late, particularly among those hoping to get in shape and burn Fat. While different weight control plans frequently set severe standards and guidelines,

16/8 irregular fasting is not difficult to follow and can give real outcomes with negligible exertion.

It's by and large thought to be not so much prohibitive, but rather more adaptable than numerous other eating regimen models and can undoubtedly find a way into pretty much any way of life. Notwithstanding upgrading weight reduction, 16/8 intermittent fasting is likewise accepted to improve glucose control, help improve brain capacity and lengthen lifespan.

Eat Stop Eat

Eat Stop Eat is an interesting way to deal with intermittent fasting that is portrayed by the consideration of up to two non-back-to-back fasting days out of each week.

For the remaining 5–6 days of the week, you can eat unreservedly. However, it's suggested that you settle on reasonable food choices and try not to eat too much. Although it appears to be illogical, you will, in any case, eat something on each scheduled day of the week when utilizing the Eat Stop Eat technique.

For example, in case you're fasting from 9 a.m. Tuesday until 9 a.m. Wednesday, you'll try to eat supper before 9 a.m. on Tuesday. Your next supper will happen after 9 a.m. on Wednesday. Thusly, you guarantee you're fasting for an entire 24 hours — yet no longer.

Remember that even on fasting long periods of Eat Stop Eat, legitimate hydration is unequivocally encouraged. Drinking a lot of water is the most ideal choice, but at the same time, you're permitted different kinds of no-calorie refreshments, for example, unsweetened espresso or tea.

12:12 Intermittent Fasting Protocol

The guidelines for this eating routine are straightforward. You must choose and stick to a 12-hour fasting window consistently. As indicated by certain analysts, fasting for 10–16 hours can make the body transform its Fat stores into energy, which discharges ketones into the circulation system. This ought to energize weight reduction. This kind of intermittent fasting plan might be a decent alternative for novices.

This is because the fasting window is generally small, a large part of the fasting happens during sleep, and the individual can devour a similar number of calories every day. The most effortless approach to do the 12-hour quickly is to remember the time of sleep is part of the fasting window.

For instance, an individual could decide to fast between 7 p.m. to 7 a.m. They would have to complete their supper before 7 p.m. also, wait until 7 a.m. to have breakfast. However, they would be snoozing for a significant part of the time in the middle.

The 14:10 Intermittent Fasting Protocol

Intermittent fasting 14:10 has an eating segment of 10 hours and a fasting segment of 14 hours. One basic way to deal with doing this is to eat regularly in the hours between 9 a.m. to 7 p.m. The timeframe between 7 p.m. to 9 a.m. the following day is the fasting window.

During the eating period, you can eat your typical suppers and snacks. Moreover, during the fasting window, you are not permitted to eat any Calories. In any case, you can drink water and unsweetened espresso or green tea.

The 20:4 Intermittent Fasting Protocol

This eating routine is viewed as a sort of intermittent fasting, an umbrella term for eating models that incorporate times of diminished calorie admission over a described period. The 20:4 is also known as the Warrior Diet, which depends on the eating examples of old heroes, who ate little during the day and afterward ate around evening time. Individuals following this eating regimen under eat for 20 hours out of every day, then devour as much food as they wanted around evening time.

During the 20-hour fasting period, health food nuts are urged to devour modest quantities of dairy items, hard-boiled eggs, and veggies, and organic foods, as well as a lot of non-calorie liquids.

Chapter 3. Tips and Tricks on Getting Started

It's Your 50s. It's time to continue being healthy. The body needs to be corrected in some way as it is entering the next stage of your life. In this part, we're going to take a look at the simple changes that are important for you to know, including what fasting can do for you.

How It Works

Fasting is a practice that almost all religions have been using for thousands of years. This means that fasting has been known for over 2,500 years now. It's safe to assume that if something has been used for this long, then it must be making some kind of difference in the lives of people who follow it. In February 2007, researchers from a group called The National Weight Control Registry (NWCR) published a study looking at 5,871 individuals who were committed to their weight loss program and followed their progress every three years over the course of 20 years.

What researchers found was that on average, the participants who were willing to develop this fasting lifestyle lost over 13 pounds in just a few weeks. Their weight overall and waist circumference also decreased by 2.3 cm overall. Fasting worked for both men and women and their weight reduction was not only proven to be safe but effective as well.

Why It's Effective

The reason why fasting works so well for so many people is that it resets the internal clock which is the timekeeper for all your body's processes; including digestion of food, regulating insulin levels in the body, etc.

Fasting resets your internal clock in a way that allows your body to burn fat at a more effective rate, and thus decreases Fat storage and the risk of developing diabetes. However, it's important to note that fasting is not something that you should be doing every day. It's actually recommended that you do it once per month, or once per season. You do get some benefits from doing this frequently, but for one month at least, you'll want to follow the recommendation of doing it once per month.

How to Do It

If you're going too fast for about 24 hours once per month, then you'll want to start with a 12 hour fast. This means that you'll only eat during the 12 hours before your usual mealtime. In addition to this, you'll want to make sure that you don't eat anything after about 18:00. This means that if you plan to eat dinner at 22:00, then don't eat anything after 18:00.

By following these tips, you'll be able to get all the benefits of fasting without having any negative side effects at all. It's important for those who are first starting out with this type of dieting technique to stop and think about what they're doing initially because anything beyond 24 hours can be dangerous and lead to some serious problems in your body.

Changing Your Diet

Changing your diet in order to make sure that you're getting the best out of your fasting is really important. As you get older, the body becomes less efficient at burning Fat. This means that it's a much better idea to change your diet than it is to rely on your body

19

changing itself. Some of the things that you'll want to start looking at are getting rid of simple starches and sugars. These foods are going to begin raising your blood sugar levels and making them difficult for your body to maintain. You'll also want to make sure that you're getting as much Fiber as you can. Fiber is going to help your digestive system, and it makes a big difference.

Beyond just changing the foods that you eat, it's also important to drink a lot of water - at least 1.5 liters per day (more if possible). Water is going to help fill your body with a liquid, and this will help flush out toxins as well. As part of this, it's also important to get enough salt in your diet. The recommended amount for adults is around 2 grams per day (more if possible), but remember that you'll need more salt during fasting than normal because, without the salt, your body can't retain any water.

In addition to not eating simple sugars and starches, it's also important to control the amount of sodium that you're getting in your diet. During normal circumstances, you should be able to get enough potassium in your diet (as long as you're eating enough vegetables). However, during fasting, you'll need more salt than normal for it to have any effect on your body. This means that instead of adding sodium to your food, you'll want to add more potassium instead. Good sources of potassium include potatoes with the skin on; bananas; tomatoes; raisins; leafy greens and broccoli.

Tricks and Tips for Staying Healthy After 50

The older you get, the more you need to take care of yourself. That means not smoking, eating right, and getting regular exercise. Improving the health of your mouth is important for preventing lots of problems like heart disease and diabetes.

It's never too late to take care of your health. If you are over 50, here are some things to think about:

- Are you drinking enough water? Staying hydrated is important. If you feel like your mouth always feels dry, you know that you aren't drinking enough of it.
- What about exercise? Bicycling is a good form of aerobic exercise that also helps to strengthen your heart muscles as well as making you breathe easily as you get older.
- Just like with the rest of your body, you want to make sure that they are healthy by doing regular dental examinations and cleanings.
- You can help prevent bone loss by taking calcium and vitamin D, as well as making sure you have enough vitamin K.
- As you get older, regular exercise is important for keeping the joints flexible as well as preventing arthritis from developing. So, make it a point to be active all the time!

Chapter 4. Shopping List to Prepare You for the Intermittent Fasting Diet

Eating during intermittent fasting (IF) can be befuddling. This is since it isn't an eating routine plan but is instead an eating strategy. We have made an intermittent fasting food list that will keep you healthy while you are on your weight reduction venture.

It tells you when to eat yet doesn't refer to what food sources can be used for your eating routine. An absence of clear dietary rules can give a false impression that one can eat anything they desire. For other people, this can cause issues with picking the "right" foods and beverages.

What to Buy:

For Protein:
- Poultry and fish

- Eggs

- Seafood

- Milk, yogurt, and cheese

- Seeds and nuts

- Beans and legumes

- Soy

- Whole grains

For veggies and other foods:
- Sweet potatoes

- Beetroots

- Quinoa

- Oats

- Brown rice

- Bananas

- Mangoes

- Apples

- Berries

- Kidney beans

- Pears

- Avocado

- Carrots

- Broccoli

- Brussels sprouts

- Almonds

- Chia seeds

- Chickpeas

For Fats:
- Avocados

- Nuts

- Cheese

- Whole eggs

- Dark chocolate

- Fatty fish

- Chia seeds

- Extra virgin olive oil (EVOO)

- Full-Fat Yogurt

For hydration:
- Water

- Sparkling water

- Black coffee or tea

- Watermelon

- Strawberries

- Cantaloupe

- Peaches

- Oranges

- Skim milk

- Lettuce

- Cucumber

- Celery

- Tomatoes

- Plain yogurt

What not to buy:

- Processed foods

- Refined grains

- Trans-Fat

- Sugar-sweetened beverages

- Candy bars

- Processed meats

- Alcoholic beverages

Foods to Eat and Avoid in Intermittent Fasting

What to Eat

Berries

Berries are very healthy, incredibly flavorful, and much lower in calories and sugar than you might think! Their tart sweetness can bring a smoothie to life, and they make a delicious snack on their own without any help from things like cream or sugar.

Cruciferous vegetables

These are vegetables like cabbage, Brussels sprouts, broccoli, and cauliflower. These are beautiful additions to your diet because they're packed with vital nutrients and with fiber that your body will love and use with a quickness!

Eggs

Eggs are such a great addition to your diet because they're packed to the gills with Protein, you can do just about anything with them, they're easy to prepare, travel well if you hard boil them, and they can pair with just about anything. They're an excellent Protein source for salads, and they're right on their own as well.

Fish

In particular, whitefish is typically very lean, but fish like salmon that have a little bit of color in them are packed with Protein, Fats, and oils that are great for you. They're good for brain and heart health, and there's a massive array of delicious things you can do with them.

Healthy starches like individual potatoes (with skins!)

In particular, red potatoes are excellent to eat, even if you're trying to lose weight because your body can use those carbs for fuel, and the skins are packed with minerals that your body will enjoy. A little bit of potato here and their can-do good things for your nutrition, but they are also a great way to feel like you're getting a little more of those fun foods that you should cut back on.

Legumes

Beans, beans, the magical fruit. They're packed with protein, and the starch in them makes them stick to your ribs without making you pay for it later. They're lovely in soups, salads, and just about any other meal of the day that you're looking to fill out. By adding beans to your regimen, you might find that your meals stick with you a little bit longer and leave you feeling more satisfied than you thought possible.

Nuts

I know you've heard people talking about how a handful of almonds makes a great snack, and if you're anything like me, you've always had kind of a hard time believing it. Nuts, as it turns out, have a good deal of their healthy Fats in them that your body can use to get through those rough patches and, while they were not the most satisfying snack on their own, you might consider topping your salad with them for a little bit of crunch, or pairing them with some berries to make them a little more satisfying.

Probiotics help boost your gut health.

Having a happy gut often means that your dietary success and overall health will improve!

Vegetables that are rich in healthy fats.

Not to sound topical or trendy, but avocados are a great example of a vegetable packed with healthy Fats. Look for vegetables with Fatty acids and a higher Fat content, and you will find that if you add more of those into your regimen, you will get hungry less often.

Water, water, water, and more water.

No matter what you decide to add to or subtract from your regimen, stay hydrated. It will help digestive health and ease, and it will keep you from feeling slump or tired, keeping you from getting too hungry. Add electrolytes where you need to, and don't be shy about bringing a bottle with you when you go from place to place. Stay hydrated!

What to Avoid

Grains

Whole grains may have their health benefits and be full of Fiber, and you can also get these nutrients elsewhere. The human diet does not require grain consumption. The truth is while grains may have some benefits, they are ridiculously high in both total and net carbohydrates, making them incompatible with the ketogenic diet.

Some people do try what is known as the targeted ketogenic diet, which is a version of the diet specifically designed for those who complete extended and strenuous workouts. With the targeted ketogenic diet, a person will consume a small serving of carb-heavy food, such as grains, for thirty to forty minutes before working out.

Starchy Vegetables and Legumes

Some vegetables are high in carbohydrates. It includes potatoes, beans, beets, corn, and more. These vegetables may have nutritional benefits, but you can get these same nutrients in low-carb vegetable alternatives.

Sugary Fruits

Most fruits contain a high sugar content, meaning that they are also high in carbohydrates. It is important to avoid most fruits. The exception is that you can enjoy berries, lemons, and limes in moderation. Some people will also enjoy a small serving of melon as a treat from time to time, but watch your portion size as it can add up quickly!

Milk and Low-Fat Dairy Products

As you can enjoy dairy products such as cheese on the ketogenic diet, you may consider trying milk. Sadly, milk is much higher in carbohydrates than cheese, with a glass of two-percent milk containing twelve Carbs, half of your daily total. Instead, choose low-carb and dairy-free milk alternatives such as almond, coconut, and soy milk.

You may consider using low-Fat cheeses instead of full Fat to reduce the saturated Fats you are consuming. The reason for this is because when the cheese is made with low-Fat dairy, it naturally has a higher carbohydrate content, which will cut into your daily net carb total.

Cashews, Pistachios, and Chestnuts

While you can enjoy nuts and seeds in moderation, keep in mind that nuts contain a moderate carbohydrate level and therefore should be eaten in moderation. However, some nuts are high in Carbs and thus are not fed on the ketogenic diet, including cashews, pistachios, and chestnuts.

If you want to enjoy nuts, you can fully enjoy almonds, pecans, walnuts, macadamia nuts, and other options instead of these options.

Most Natural Sweeteners

While you can undoubtedly enjoy sugar-free natural sweeteners such as stevia, monk fruit, and sugar alcohols, you should avoid natural sweeteners that contain sugar. Suffice to say, and the sugar content makes these sweeteners naturally high in Carbs. But, not only that, but they will also spike your blood sugar and insulin. It means you should avoid things such as honey, agave, maple, coconut palm sugar, and dates.

Alcohol

Alcohol is not generally enjoyed on the ketogenic diet, as your body will be unable to burn off Calories while your liver attempts to process alcohol. Many people also find that when they are in ketosis, they get drunk more quickly and experience more severe hangovers. Not only that, but alcohol adds unnecessary Calories and carbohydrates to your diet.

The worst offenders to choose would be margaritas, piña coladas, sangrias, Bloody Mary, whiskey sours, cosmopolitans, and regular beers.

But, if you choose to drink alcohol regardless of drink in moderation and choose low-carb versions such as rum, vodka, tequila, whiskey, and gin. The next-best options would be dry wines and light beers.

Chapter 5. Mistakes to Avoid in Intermittent Fasting

The results of intermittent fasting vary from one person to the other, but overall, every individual should be able to reap some benefits from the fasting. The key is doing it right, and doing it consistently. Here are some common mistakes that could compromise your outcome:

Starting with an Extreme Plan

Now that you have found a fasting plan that sounds just perfect for your needs, don't you just want to jump in there with all your enthusiasm and, well, kick the hell out of it? You must be already imagining your new look after shedding those extra pounds. Can the fasting start already? Well, not so fast. Don't let your zest lead you to an intense plan which will subject your body to a drastic change. You can't come from 3 meals a day and snacks in between to a 24 hour fast. That will only leave you feeling miserable. Start with skipping single meals. Or avoiding snacks. Once your body gets used to short fasts, you can proceed to as far as your body can take, within reasonable limits. Go slow on exercising as well during the fasting phase, at least in the initial weeks, as it could cause Adrenal Fatigue.

Quitting Too Soon

Have you been fasting for a paltry one week and have already decided that it is too hard? Are you struggling with hunger pangs, cravings, mood swings, low energy levels and so on? Well, such a reaction should be anticipated. The first couple of weeks can be harsh as the body adjusts to the reduced calorie intake. You will be hungry, irritable and exhausted. Still, you will be required to remain consistent. Even if you cannot feel it, the body is adapting to the changes. If you give up during this period and revert to normal eating, you'll just roll back on the adjustments that the body had already made. Any change requires discipline, and this one is no exception. Hang in there; things will get better with time.

'Feasting' Too Much

Some quarters refer to intermittent fasting as alternating phases of fasting and feasting. This largely suggests that as soon as the clock hits the last minute of fast time, you dig right into a large savory meal, the kind that you end with a loud satisfied belch. Ideally, there should be nothing wrong with this approach, after all, you've successfully made it through your fasting window.

But remember your main goal here is to burn fat and lose weight. That only works if you have fewer Calories going in compared to those going out. The larger your meal, the higher the number of calories that you're introducing into the body.

You don't need to eat a mountain. Start with fruits and vegetables. They contain Fiber that will leave you feeling fuller, so you won't need that large of a meal. Eat slowly, listening to the signals of getting full. Stop eating as soon as you feel full, even if there's still food on your plate, which you may have piled up due to the hunger you were feeling. Refrigerate the extra for another meal. You don't have to eat all through the eating window either. Once you're satisfied, go on and concentrate on other things.

Insufficient Calories

While some will binge eat to make up for the 'lost time,' others will eat very little, fearing to turn back the gains already made. This results in inadequate Calories, yet these Calories are required to fuel the body to perform its functions optimally. With insufficient nutrients, you're likely to experience mood swings, irritability, fatigue, and low energy levels. Your day-to-day life will be compromised, and you'll be less productive. Intermittent fasting should make your life better, not worse. Eating enough will allow you to remain active, and proceed efficiently with your fasting plan.

Wrong Food Choices

We have already established that intermittent fasting concentrates largely on the when as opposed to what regarding eating. While that still leaves an opportunity to enjoy a wide variety of foods, it does not mean that you can eat whatever you want. Left to our own devices, most of us will go for sugary and fatty foods as they're very enticing to the taste buds. French fries, pizza, cake, cookies, candy, ice cream, processed meats and so on. This is a very short-sighted approach though. Breaking your fast with such foods will only erase the benefits of the fast.

Go for healthy, wholesome foods that will nourish your body with all groups of nutrients. Let your meal contain adequate portions of vegetables, protein, good fats and complex carbs. You may have heard that intermittent fasting works well with a low-carb diet. That's right, but it's a low-carb, not a no-carb diet. Some people try to accelerate weight loss by eliminating all Carbs. Remember Carbs supply us with Calories to fuel the body. Include a portion of healthy starch on your plate, going for brown unprocessed options where applicable.

Why should you worry about what you eat yet intermittent fasting is about when you eat? Well, healthy eating is for everyone, even if you're not going through a fasting plan. You eat wholesome foods because they're good for the body, and they keep you away from lifestyle diseases. Healthy eating should be normal eating, so in this case, we can agree that the fast is accompanied by normal eating.

Insufficient Fluids

Staying hydrated makes your fast more tolerable. It provides you a full feeling and retains hunger pangs at bay. Fasting also breaks down the damaged components in the body, and the water helps flush them out as toxins.

You can also sip tea or coffee, with no milk or sugar added. Coffee has been known to contain compounds that further accelerate the burning of fat. Green tea also has similar properties. You can test with diverse flavors of tea or coffee to get a taste that appeals to you. As long as they don't contain any calories, they're good to go.

Over-Concentrating on the Eating Window

If you can't take your eyes off the clock, you're not doing it right. You can't spend the fasting phase obsessing over food, thinking of what and how much you'll eat when it's finally time. In fact, the more you think about food, the hungrier you get. That hunger you feel every 5 hours or so is emotional hunger. It is clock hunger, which you'll feel around the normal mealtimes. Real hunger mostly checks in when you've been fasting for 16 hours onwards. Get your mind off food and concentrate on something else. If you're at home and keep circling the kitchen, leave and go somewhere else. Go to the library, for shopping (not for food of course), to the park or attend to your errands. Food is so much easier to keep away from when it's out of sight.

Wrong Plan

We have already been through the various fasting plans available, as well as the factors to consider when choosing a fasting plan. That should guide you to comfortable fasting. How do you know that the plan your following is not the best one for you? To begin with, the entire process becomes a major strain. You struggle with hunger, Fatigue, mood swings, and low energy levels. Your performance in your duties is affected, and you dread the next fast. And even after all the struggle, there's hardly any significant result to show for it. Go back and study the plans and choose one that better suits your lifestyle.

Stress

If you're under a great deal of stress, chances are you'll struggle through the fast. Stress causes hormone imbalances leaving you struggling with hunger pangs when you should have been fasting comfortably. Stress eating is common, characterized by cravings that drive you towards fatty and sugary foods. It also interferes with sleep, and fasting is even harder when you're not well-rested. If you've already attempted the fast and have fallen into any of these mistakes, as many often do, you can correct yourself and proceed. If you're just starting out, you now know the pitfalls to avoid. The key is to keep learning and improving, and the results will be a testament to your effort.

Managing Stress

Now that we've established that stress is one of the factors that can impair your fasting, it is imperative that you learn how to manage stress.

Here are some steps that you can take to ensure that stress does not hinder you from healthy living:

Relax Daily

Those issues that you carry in your heart and mind can cause you to get stressed in the long run. Find a way to unwind at the end of every day so that the pressure does not build up. Watch a movie, sport, documentary, read a book, try a new recipe, soak in the bathtub or do whatever else entertains you. Those few hours provide a positive distraction so that you can face the following day without tagging along with yesterday's challenges.

Open Up

Let somebody else know what is going on. A problem shared is half solved. Just speaking out makes you feel lighter even before you find a solution. Stress can prejudice your reasoning and judgment, making it difficult to evaluate the issues you're facing. Someone else, looking at your situation with a rational eye, will be better placed to assess the situation and suggest solutions. Speak to a family member, friend or colleague. If you feel the matter is too personal and you prefer to speak to an expert, there are counselors available.

Get a Hobby

What is it that you enjoy doing? That thing that commands your undivided attention for hours? It could be cycling, gardening, drawing, painting, cooking, video games and so on. Give it more time and attention. Set yourself new goals. For instance, you could challenge yourself to finish a drawing in a week. Or grow a vegetable patch in a month. Or knit a sweater in 3 days. Or try out a new recipe every evening.

With a goal comes commitment. Now your mind will be shifted from the issues causing you stress to something new and exciting. With every goal achieved comes a sense of accomplishment, further improving your mood. Interact with others who have a similar hobby. Join a relevant community. Even an online one will do. Take part in their activities. No matter what you're going through on any day, you have something to look forward to.

Enough Sleep

The relationship between stress and sleep is an awkward one. You're required to have enough sleep to better manage stress, yet the stress itself keeps you from sleeping. You have to look for a different trigger for sleep. Read a book, listen to music, take a relaxing shower, or whatever else soothes you to sleep. When well-rested, you'll be better placed to evaluate the causes of your stress and possibly come up with possible solutions.

We've just spoken about making changes, right? Perhaps one of those changes that you need to make is to deactivate/suspend your account and leave the inter-web for some time. Figure out your life without all the senseless pressure. Deal with people that you can show the real you and they support you. Build your life quietly and consistently. As they say, work quietly and let success make the noise.

These tips should help you control or even eliminate your stress, and you can then fast without strain.

Chapter 6. Best Exercises and Lifestyle in Weight Loss

Physical activity is the last piece of the weight loss triad, but it is in no way less important. Exercising gets your blood pumping, releases endorphins after and during workouts, and may help you burn extra calories. The number of calories you burn will depend on the type of exercise, duration, and intensity. However, this is generally a small amount and is nowhere near the number of calories you burn from the basal metabolic rate. The average Joe will not have the time or resources to devote significant attention to burning Calories. Instead, exercise helps in other ways. In the case of intermittent fasting, it can help regulate your energy levels and deplete available glycogen stores, forcing your body to burn fat if it isn't already. Remember those old-school workout videos with everyone talking about "feeling the burn?" Very rarely will exercise directly burn Fat. In fact, Fat only gets burned after glycogen stores are gone (which takes a while). Most amateur athletes never get to that level of performance. We sometimes hear that burning x amounts of Calories (3,500, for example) equals burning 1 pound of Fat. More specifically, you are burning 3,500 Calories, which results in losing one pound of Fat, more or less.

Many people feel that exercising on an empty stomach is bad for you. One way this could be true is by causing a significant drop in blood sugar levels. Here, diabetics need to be extra careful. The best time for them to exercise would be just hours after starting a fast—when food energy is still running high in the body. An exercise of any kind will naturally bring blood sugar levels down. If someone can't regulate blood sugar levels efficiently (diabetes) they run the danger of having a serious episode of low blood sugar. Otherwise, the body can detect that blood sugar levels are dropping and make an adequate response to metabolize glycogen. People who find it difficult to exercise while fasting may elect to "cheat" by having a small meal prior to the workout. Protein shakes are notorious for this, as they tend to be high in both carbohydrates and Proteins. Mixing whey Protein with water may run anywhere between 120 and 400 Calories depending on how much powder is used. Mixing it with milk will increase the calorie content significantly. But normally Protein shakes aren't required to get through exercise.

If you are already acclimatized to the Fat-burning stage of a low-carb diet, you will find it easier to get through regular exercise even when fasted. Trying to get a full workout in during the first week of Keto will prove difficult. Trying to exercise in the middle of a fast is also hard because you will suffer from the symptoms of low blood sugar. Diabetics will need to take precautions against them. Since a diabetic should be monitoring blood sugar levels regularly, they should schedule a blood meter test shortly before deciding to exercise.

The types of exercise you decide on undertaking will depend on your fitness goals. A good general recommendation for people who wish to be healthier is resistance training at least two times a week alongside the recommended 150 minutes a week of moderate to intense aerobic activity. These 150 minutes can further be increased to 300 minutes to receive even more benefits. These include lowering the risk of cardiovascular disease, reduction of the risk of cancers, and a greater increase in weight-loss potential from physical activity alone. Whether a full 300 minutes of exercise is sustainable a week while fasting will depend on the fitness level of the person, as well as what their fasting routines look like—for example, somebody who is doing the "5:2" Method may simply decide not to exercise on their fasting days. Others who fast daily by skipping breakfast (and fasting overnight) may decide to get the workout done after the fasting period is over. Breaking the fast with a small meal and then doing the workout afterward is a good option. Exercise gets a little trickier on those longer (1–3 days or more) fasts. The considerations are still the same and the risk of a low blood sugar episode increases.

Benefits of Exercising While Fasted

While you can expect working out on an empty stomach to be a challenge, there are many benefits to be had. First, working out with no food in your system means that Calories expended directly take a hit to your glycogen stores. In the short term, this means that you will lose weight quickly from the water stored in glycogen and may accelerate Fat burning. Along with burning the glycogen, you can expect cellular processes to burn at least some Fat. There are called AMP kinases and are responsible for jump-starting Fat metabolism in muscles during workouts. They only burn Fat when the body detects that there isn't enough caloric energy to go around from glucose. The real nitty-gritty of what happens during exercise while fasted can get complicated fast, but your body secretes all sorts of things. Muscles that are exposed to undue oxidative stress from exercising while fasted become resilient to such stress over time, preventing the pace of the aging process. The brain and muscle tissues enter a rejuvenation process similar to autophagy that keeps things running smoothly. These effects are mostly stimulated during short, intense workouts like HIT workouts and resistance training.

Small amounts of human growth hormone (HGH) are also released if you exercise when glucose stores are low. In turn, this stimulates the secretion of androgens like testosterone that fuel libido and increase lean muscle mass.

Aerobic Exercise

Anything that gets you moving around is considered aerobic. In specific, it deals with raising your heart rate for extended periods of time. It comes from the word that means "with oxygen," causing you to breathe faster than usual while giving your body enough oxygen to flow in the blood. Walking, jogging, jump rope, cycling, stair climbing, and countless sports all qualify for aerobic exercise. Current American physical activity guidelines recommend at least 150 minutes of this type of exercise a week. One of the easiest things you can do is walk. Walking is virtually free in most cases and can be a pleasant change of pace. You can take your dog or a buddy along with you to keep you company.

Aerobic exercise while fasted will use glycogen primarily as fuel, depending on how far into the fast you are. If you exercise just after your last meal, you can get an energy boost from that. Believe it or not, people who work out on their fasting period report higher levels of energy they do during non-fasted workouts. This has primarily to do with the body's secretion of HGH, among other things to compensate for the lack of readily available energy. But these levels of energy are usually reserved for people who are used to fasting. If you try to exercise during your first weeks of trying it out, expect major resistance from your body. It is advisable to take things slow and to increase the intensity or duration of fasted workouts gradually. You can exercise on non-fasting days as usual.

Anaerobic Exercise

The opposite of aerobic exercise is the anaerobic kind. This covers different forms of resistance training, including bodyweight exercises, strength conditioning, and weight lifting. Also covered here are high-intensity workouts like HIT and sprints training. Anaerobic exercise and resistance training, in general, are good for creating muscle and strengthening bones. The nervous system also benefits from the mind-body connection used with resistance training. Resistance is effectively teaching the muscles how to interface with signals from

41

the brain. Both anaerobic and aerobic exercise should be used together to get maximum weight loss results.

The difference between them is that under anaerobic conditions the oxygen that enters the body through the lungs is not enough energy to sustain the workout. Instead, muscles need to break down sugars (glycogen) to get the energy they need. This breakdown facilitates weight loss by reducing the amount of available glycogen at a given time. Broken down glycogen stores are converted into lactic acid buildup—the primary reason why muscles feel sore following an intense workout.

The breakdown of muscles also elicits a repair mechanism not only to mend torn muscle Fibers but to flush out dead components from cells. You should instantly recognize this as autophagy. You will experience a boost in metabolism that lasts hours after your workout, whether you are in a fasting state or not.

Working with the Fast, Not Against It

The base rule for working out while fasting is not to push things. If you at any time feel dizzy, get migraines, start vomiting, etc. in the middle of the workout, it is not a challenge to push yourself forward, but a sign that you need to stop.

Hydration is important, as dehydration is a leading cause of heatstroke. If you plan on lifting heavy weights for anaerobic exercise, make sure you work with a lighter weight than usual during fasting days. Lifting heavy with insufficient glycogen stores is a good way to pass out in front of everyone at the gym. Not fun.

Chapter 7. How to Determine Excess Weight?

Weight Index isn't just about the amount you weigh, yet in addition, it mulls over your height.

You should determine your Body Mass Index (BMI) to see whether you're qualified for a medical procedure.

The Body Mass Index is your weight in kilograms partitioned by the square of your stature in meters. You might be qualified if your BMI is more than 40 (sullen stoutness) or more than 35 with a genuine heftiness-related wellbeing condition, for example, uncontrolled Type 2 diabetes, rest apnea, or extreme joint torment that restricts your everyday exercises.

Understanding Weight Reduction Measurements

Utilizing the measurements of Excess Body Weight and Excess Weight Loss (EWL) encourages us to see how much weight reduction we should anticipate with relation to our height.

You may hear that somebody has shed 50 pounds, yet without ascertaining their EBW and EWL there is no chance to determine whether they have lost a ton or a little measure of weight comparative with their body height. On the off chance that the individual who shed those 50 pounds is taller than you and has several pounds more to lose than you, 50 pounds isn't that much weight to lose. Nonetheless, if the individual just had 50 pounds to lose, we can affirm that the individual lost 100 percent EWL and has arrived at their weight reduction target!

Pounds

In the UK it is standard to quantify body weight in pounds. For example, an individual gauging 250 pounds may have a goal of shedding 100 pounds to arrive at a goal weight of 150 pounds. When estimating weight reduction utilizing BMI measurements it is essential to contrast weight, weight loss goals, and height. Therefore, Excess Body Weight and Excess Weight Loss are frequently utilized.

Overabundance Body Weight

EBW is the measure of body weight you have in an overabundance of your goal weight. The ordinary BMI is around 24. The perfect body weight for an individual of a height of 5 feet 7 inches is around 150 pounds.

Overabundance Weight Loss

EWL is the level of your EBW that you lose. We figure EWL by separating the number of pounds lost by the measure of pounds in your EBW. For instance, if your EBW is 100 pounds and you shed 45 pounds, your EWL is 45
percent.

The scale? It the DEVIL!

Well, pause. Give me a chance to qualify for that announcement. In the event that the scale is tumbling in a descending movement, demonstrating to you steady and great loss for quite a while, consistently, without interference, at that point the scale most likely isn't the DEVIL to you.

Go figure

In any case, I'm not here to persuade you to surrender the scale. That may cause a revolt and honestly, I don't have a home security framework. Rather, I need to urge you to take a gander at a few unique measurements to keep tabs on your development rather than just taking a gander at the scale.

What Is % Excess Body Weight Loss?

One measure to think about is your% Body Weight Loss Abundance. That is actually what it seems like. It's the level of the measure of weight you need to lose, that you have just lost. (Do those words sound as tangled to you as they do to me?)

We intermittently check our % EBW (as I call it for short). Each time I do it, individuals get so upbeat. This number makes you feel way superior to the scale since it shows that you are so near to where you need to be. It disposes of all that "Is 150 lbs. extremely thin... or should I go for 130?" business. It disposes of the "X, Y and Z lost 7,085 lbs. their initial two weeks after a medical procedure and I'm in a slowdown!" business. It focuses on you and your progress and shows you how far you have come.

Chapter 8. FAQ About Intermittent Fasting

- Can I Have Coffee?
- Truly, you can have a dark espresso, water, and plain tea
- Can I Add Cream/Sugar/Milk to My Coffee?

The objective of fasting isn't to add Calories, so the appropriate response is no; you ought not to add anything to your espresso. Nonetheless, I have known about cases in which intermittent fasters add under 50 Calories to their espresso. They have professed to be effective with intermittent fasting; I have heard that it doesn't influence their abstained state; however, remember all people are most certainly not the same. I would not prescribe adding anything to your espresso, yet if adding something to your espresso makes this a good chance for the objective you have for yourself, at that point, check it out.

- Does Intermittent Fasting Work Well with Veganism, Paleo, Keto, Vegetarianism, or Any Other Styles of Eating?

Indeed, the magnificence of intermittent fasting is that it tends to be joined with any way of eating except if coordinated by a clinical expert. You can transform your way of eating into the 16:8 technique effortlessly, as this change does not limit or express the style/sorts of food you eat; it is explicitly founded on the condition of your eating.

- Is There an Alternative to the 16:8 Method If I Cannot Initially Fast 16 Hours and Want to Work My Way Up to 16?

Yes, particularly for ladies, it is suggested that if ladies can't or are not ready to do a 16-hour quick, they can begin with a 14-hour fasting window also, a 10-hour eating window. This is suggested for ladies; however, men can start here if necessary. When the 14 hours are dominated, you would then be able to work your way up to the 16:8 strategy.

- Can I Have a Cheat Meal?

You can eat what you want when intermittent fasting; there are no nutritional category limitations. There is no cheat meal to have except if you have concluded that you have put yourself on some prohibitive dinners/food sources to not enjoy; provided that this is true, at that point truly, however, I suggest consistently to eat with some restraint.

- What Are Some Healthy Snack Foods to Eat on the Go During My Feeding Window?

Pepperoni cuts, organic products, veggie plate, Skinny Pop popcorn in singular packs (except if you will consistently gauge the servings before burning-through), turkey/meat jerky, singular peanut butter cups, whole grain oats, almond milk, eggs, rice cakes, nuts (singular packs), hummus, and that's only the beginning.

- I Am Too Hungry During My Fasting Window; What Should I Do?

Be patient, and trust that your body will adjust to this change. This may take some time; for a few, it happens quickly; for other people, it might require a week or somewhere in the vicinity, yet this relies upon how you were eating before beginning this way of life. Concurring to Collier in 2013, your body is as yet changing by how it was working previously and is battling you to return to that way, as a great many people were eating too much and perhaps more dinners or snacks during the day. Ultimately, you won't feel along these lines. Eventually, you will adjust to your eating and fasting windows, and the urge to eat or the prospect of starving will decrease until it disappears.

- Why Am I Not Losing Fat Faster, Like Other People Are?

It is without a doubt a mix of not eating the appropriate bits at the point when you are eating or potentially not planning to eat the correct food choices. Albeit Fat and weight reduction can, in any case, occur, it's more successive and noticeable at the point when the suitable food choices and portions are chosen and planned.

- How Can I Stay Full Longer?

Stay hydrated and eat food enriched in Fiber.

- Do I Have to Eat Low Carb?

No, you can eat what you want during your eating window. I suggest eating proportionately and picking on better food choices. Rather than white bread, pick whole grain bread. Rather than white rice, pick brown rice. Rather than anything with high fructose corn syrup, scratch it off; rather than a canned organic product, eat the natural product.

- Should I Exercise in the Fasted State?

It's not mandatorily required to lift heavy weights, but you can do normal day-to-day exercise like running, walking, or stretching.

- What If I Am on Medications and Must Eat with My Morning Medications?

In this situation, make sure that your feeding time matches with your medication time. In this case, you would need to make your feeding window begin at whatever time you take your meds. I would

48

recommend taking your meds as late as you can in the mornings, but do get authorization of your plan from a medical professional.

- Should I Deliberate This with My Medical Professional Before Beginning the Change?
- Truly, you ought to consistently examine diet changes with a clinical expert before you start.
- Why Should One Start Intermittent Fasting?

The main explanation behind beginning this eating regimen plan is to get thinner without changing one's eating routine to an extraordinary level. With this eating routine plan, you are allowed to maintain your body's bulk and stay slender. This is conceivable since, in such a case, that lessens midsection Fat as the eating routine advances. This diet plan requires little change and no convoluted schedules.

- Is Skipping Breakfast Considered Unhealthy for the Body?

This is a myth that a great many people consider as being valid. This generalization should be evaded. Some say that getting up and eating assists the body with getting the energy it needs for the entire day. That may be valid, yet if you are following a solid eating regimen for the remainder of your meals, skipping breakfast ought not to affect your way of life. It may require some investment to become accustomed to avoiding a meal after you awaken with an empty stomach, yet that will help the absorptive state occur to detoxify the body and clean your internal organs.

- Is It Okay to Take Supplements with an Intermittent Fasting Regimen?

Of course, you can take those supplements but do not forget to check the side effects. Some of them may work in a way that is better than others. For example, Fat-dissolvable vitamins will be more powerful with your meals during eating hours. Pick them over other kinds of supplements.

- Will Intermittent Fasting Affect One's Metabolism?

Intermittent fasting favors short-term fasting goals. It won't affect your metabolism as the fasting timeframe precise.

- Can a Child Fast?

No, it would be an impractical notion for a youngster to fast. Skipping breakfast can cause an absence of growth compounds in a kid's body, and the person may not grow normally. The youngster may likewise need legitimate brain work if the individual in question follows intermittent fasting for a delayed period.

Chapter 9. Benefits of Intermittent Fasting

Lifestyle Benefits

When compared to other diets, the simplicity of intermittent fasting makes it perhaps the easiest eating protocol through which to experience significant health benefits. Often, the complexity of some eating plans causes people to fail at the first hurdle because as much as they think they understand what they should be doing, they really don't. This results in people going to punishing extremes in order to fulfill what they think they are supposed to be doing and ending up with very disappointing results. Intermittent fasting couldn't be simpler—now you eat and now you don't. Often, special diets can be extremely expensive to follow. You have to purchase special ingredients and eat food that you ordinarily wouldn't. Intermittent fasting is different in that regard too. It costs you absolutely nothing to practice intermittent fasting, and other than a caloric reduction in the case of weight loss and eating as healthy as possible, there is no dictation as to what to eat.

Intermittent fasting is flexible, so it allows you gaps in between to eat the things you enjoy. What is life without an occasional dessert, some chocolate, or pizza? With intermittent fasting, you can have those treats and not feel guilty because when you fast, your body will be burning that treat off. Of course, that is not to say that in every eating window you can binge on every fast food known to mankind. You will still need to eat a healthy diet; you just won't be weighing food and calculating its calorie content all the time.

If you have found an eating plan that you enjoy such as Keto, Paleo, or the like, you can incorporate that with intermittent fasting. There are no other plans available where you can combine two and get even better results. Intermittent fasting is a fantastic addition to other eating plans and does not detract from any other diets (Fung, 2020).

For women over 50, the adjustment to menopause can mean a temporary change in lifestyle. In severe situations, menopause can result in difficulties in relationships with partners and loved ones. Intermittent fasting can help make a big difference in these challenges, and this can be life-changing.

Health Benefits

Cardiovascular health should be a strong focus for people of all ages but even more so for women over 50. The most significant cause of death for women over 50 today is cardiovascular disease. This umbrella term describes all diseases of the heart or the arteries leading to and from the heart. This could include blockages, damage, and deformities in the structure.

The most impactful factor where diet is concerned is the types of Protein sources that are eaten as well as the types of Fats that are consumed. Plant Proteins such as beans and legumes have been proven to be a healthier source of Protein than animal Proteins in general.

Where animal Protein is concerned, the leaner the source, the better, and poultry and fish are always healthier options than red meat. The Fat component of red meat is another problem where heart disease is concerned, as are other sources of Fat such as cooking oils and spreads used for bread. Saturated Fats are the types of Fats we want to avoid in our diet, and these include animal Fat, lard, and tropical oils such as palm oil. Unsaturated Fats in small quantities are healthier. Examples of unsaturated fats include avocados, nuts, olive oil, and vegetable oils. When we eat foods in excess of what our body is able to burn, the leftover food forms triglycerides that, at high levels, contribute to the occurrence of cardiovascular disease. When we fast, our body burns triglycerides for energy thereby reducing the levels in our blood and, in turn, reducing our risk of cardiovascular disease.

In our eating window, we experience an increase in insulin levels, and when we fast, those levels are decreased. This decrease in insulin results in less food being stored as Fat. In animal trials, intermittent fasting has been shown to prevent and reverse Type 2 Diabetes. Another thing that happens when insulin levels decrease is that the FOXO transcription factors, which are known to positively impact metabolism, become more active in the body. This process is also linked to improved longevity and healthy aging.

Another no communicable disease that seems to be impacted by intermittent fasting is cancer. Growth Factor 1 (GF1) is a hormone very similar in nature to insulin, and the presence of this hormone is known to be a marker for cancer development. Levels of GF1 are reduced during intermittent fasting. Women over 50 are twice as likely to develop breast cancer, for instance, and risk factors for other common cancers are also thought to increase when women start to experience the hormonal changes of menopause. Intermittent fasting is, therefore, an excellent preventative measure for the occurrence of cancer in women over 50.

The increased cell resilience is seen in people who regularly fast has been linked to a stronger immune system as well as a general faster recovery from illness. The process of building cell resilience through fasting is similar to exercising muscles. The more you undertake regular exercise with periods of rest in between, the stronger your muscles become.

The autophagy process that is triggered by intermittent fasting has been shown to help reduce inflammation in the body as well as oxidative stress, which is primarily responsible for cell damage in the body. Inflammation in various parts of the body has been shown to be present as a precursor to the diagnosis of many different no communicable diseases. The diagnosis of no communicable diseases is far more common in women over 50 than any other age group. It is, therefore, vital for women in this age group to make use of intermittent fasting and autophagy as an additional preventative measure against the development of no communicable diseases.

The Circadian Cycle is the name given to the rhythm created in our body by light and dark (day and night). This natural rhythm controls our need to sleep and eat and has a major impact on our metabolism, cognitive function, and emotional health. It is our internal clock, and when disrupted, it can have devastating effects on our bodies. Intermittent fasting has been shown to help regulate the Circadian Cycle and, if it is out of the loop, reset it back to its natural function.

From an evolutionary perspective, our bodies are designed to eat during the day and not to eat at night. This, of course, is the reverse in certain nocturnal mammals who have evolved to reverse that Circadian Cycle due to the availability of prey at night. As modern humans, we have disrupted our Circadian Cycle by not going to sleep when the sun goes down and also continuing to eat well into the night. This impacts our metabolism and our sleeping patterns, resulting in weight gain and sleep disorders such as insomnia. By using intermittent fasting to reset our internal clock to its evolutionary default, we can encourage weight loss by optimizing our metabolism and have a more restful sleep.

In women over 50, this is particularly beneficial. As we age, sleep disorders become more common. We feel tired earlier, experience disturbed sleep, and generally find that we are unable to sleep for as many hours as we once could. This disruption in sleep, of course, has a major impact on our health both physically and mentally. The reason for this change in sleep is due to the reduced levels of Human Growth Hormone (HGH) in our bodies as we age. As we now know, intermittent fasting helps to increase the levels of HGH in our body, thus allowing us to regain a more regular sleeping pattern.

It is important to point out that your last meal of the day should be eaten at least two hours before you go to sleep, and it should be a satisfying but not overly large meal. If you eat too long before you go to bed, you may experience hunger pangs while you sleep that disrupt your sleep. The importance of a good sleeping pattern cannot be understated as poor sleeping patterns have even been shown to increase the likelihood of the occurrence of certain cancers.

Intermittent fasting has also been shown to improve the regulation of genes that promote liver health and also in the balance of gut bacteria. Gut bacteria play a role in our immune system, and it is vital to keep these gut guests in good shape to optimize your body's defense systems (Kresser, 2019).

Cognitive Functioning Benefits

As you move into your 50s, there are several different effects on your brain health and, as a result, your cognitive functioning. Brain shrinkage automatically occurs as we age, and although it is not something we can avoid, it is certainly something that we can delay and slow down. From a fasting perspective, the process of autophagy, which speeds up during fasting, can help to consume damaged brain cells and use that cellular material to produce new brain cells. This process can help to alleviate the natural brain shrinkage process.

The release of ketones during the burning of Fat which occurs during fasting is also highly beneficial to brain health. The enhanced level of ketones helps to protect the brain from the development of epileptic seizures, Alzheimer's disease, and other neurodegenerative diseases. Of course, as we age, we are also more likely to develop neurodegenerative diseases. Diseases like Alzheimer's and other forms of dementia do have a wide range of risk factors including genetics and smoking. Fasting to enhance autophagy and ketone production is one way that we put up a line of defense against these diseases.

A study conducted on participants over 50, all of whom were already exhibiting some form of impaired cognitive function, showed that by increasing the levels of ketones in the participants' bodies, their cognitive functioning increased within six weeks. It is believed that the reason ketones are so beneficial in increasing cognitive function is due to the fact that they trigger the release of brain-derived neurotrophic factor (BDNF). BDNF helps to strengthen the neural connections in our brain, which are the pathways that our brain uses to transmit thoughts and instructions. BDNF particularly helps to strengthen the pathways that focus on memory and learning. Studies have also shown that intermittent fasting also helps to promote the growth of new nerve cells in the brain.

Intermittent fasting can also help to improve neuroplasticity, which is the brain's natural capability to build new neural pathways. This is imperative in learning as well as in the breaking of habits. When we break bad habits, we actually work to remove the brain's reliance on a commonly used neural pathway and promote the use of a new pathway. Studies in people with brain injuries have shown that intermittent fasting speeds up healing.

Chapter 10. Appetizers, Sides, and Snacks

1. Roasted Brussels Sprouts with Pecans and Gorgonzola

Preparation Time: 10 minutes

Cooking Time: 35 minutes

Servings: 4

Ingredients:

- 1 lb. Brussels sprouts, fresh
- ¼ cup pecans, chopped
- 1 tbsp. olive oil
- Extra olive oil to oil the baking tray
- Pepper and salt for tasting
- ¼ cup Gorgonzola cheese (If you prefer not to use the Gorgonzola cheese, you can toss the Brussels sprouts when hot, with 2 tablespoons of butter instead.

Directions:
1. Warm the oven to 350°F or 175°C.

2. Rub a large pan or any vessel you wish to use with a little bit of olive oil. You can use a paper towel or a pastry brush.

3. Cut off the ends of the Brussels sprouts if you need to and then cut them in a lengthwise direction into halves. (Fear not if a few of the leaves come off of them, some may become deliciously crunchy during cooking).

4. Chop up all of the pecans using a knife and then measure them for the amount.

5. Put your Brussels sprouts as well as the sliced pecans inside a bowl, and cover them all with some olive oil, pepper, and salt (be generous).

6. Arrange all of your pecans and Brussels sprouts onto your roasting pan in a single layer.

7. Roast this for 30 to 35 minutes, or when they become tender and can be pierced with a fork easily. Stir during cooking if you wish to get a more even browning.

8. Once cooked, toss them with the Gorgonzola Cheese (or butter) before you serve them. Serve them hot.

Nutrition:

- Calories: 149
- Fat: 11 grams,
- Carbohydrates: 10 grams,
- Fiber: 4 grams,
- Protein: 5 grams

2. Artichoke Petals Bites

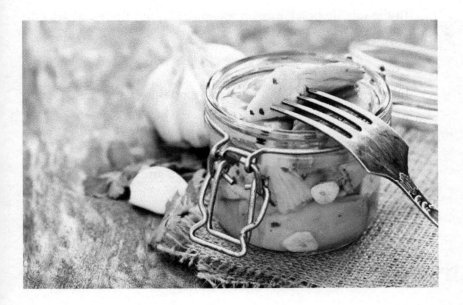

Preparation Time: 10 minutes

Cooking Time: 10 minutes

Servings: 8

Ingredients:

- 8 oz. artichoke petals, boiled, drained, without salt
- ½ cup almond flour
- 4 oz. Parmesan, grated
- 2 tbsp. almond butter, melted

Directions:

1. In the mixing bowl, mix up together almond flour and grated Parmesan.
2. Preheat the oven to 355°F.
3. Dip the artichoke petals in the almond butter and then coat in the almond flour mixture.
4. Place them in the tray.
5. Transfer the tray to the preheated oven and cook the petals for 10 minutes.
6. Chill the cooked petal bites a little before serving.

Nutrition:

- Calories: 93,
- Protein: 6.54 grams,
- Fat: 3.72 grams,
- Carbohydrates: 9.08 grams

3. Stuffed Beef Loin in Sticky Sauce

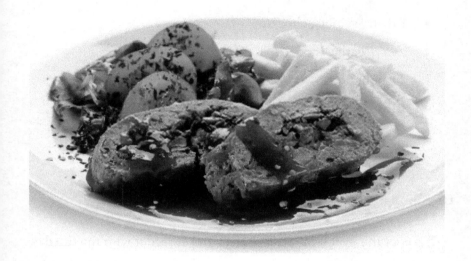

Preparation Time: 15 minutes

Cooking Time: 6 minutes

Servings: 4

Ingredients:

- 1 tbsp. Erythritol
- 1 tbsp. lemon juice
- 4 tbsp. water
- 1 tbsp. butter
- ½ tsp. tomato sauce
- ¼ tsp. dried rosemary

- 9 oz. beef loin
- 3 oz. celery root, grated
- 3 oz. bacon, sliced
- 1 tbsp. walnuts, chopped
- ¾ tsp. garlic, diced
- 2 tsp. butter
- 1 tbsp. olive oil
- 1 tsp. salt
- ½ cup of water

Directions:

1. Cut the beef loin into the layer and spread it with the dried rosemary, butter, and salt. Then place over the beef loin: grated celery root, sliced bacon, walnuts, and diced garlic.
2. Roll the beef loin and brush it with olive oil. Secure the meat with the help of the toothpicks. Place it in the tray and add a ½ cup of water.
3. Cook the meat in the preheated to 365°F oven for 40 minutes.
4. Meanwhile, make the sticky sauce.
5. Mix up together Erythritol, lemon juice, 4 tablespoons of water, and butter.
6. Preheat the mixture until it starts to boil. Then add tomato sauce and whisk it well.
7. Bring the sauce to a boil and remove it from the heat.

8. When the beef loin is cooked, remove it from the oven and brush it with the cooked sticky sauce very generously.

9. Slice the beef roll and sprinkle with the remaining sauce.

Nutrition:

- Calories: 321,
- Protein: 18.35 grams,
- Fat: 26.68 grams,
- Carbohydrates: 2.75 grams

4. Eggplant Fries

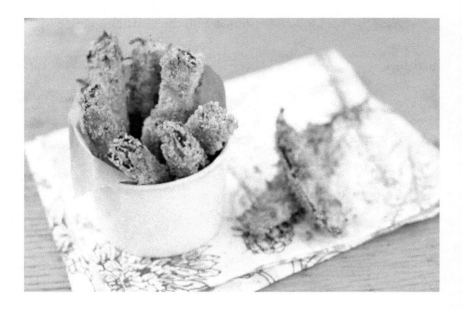

Preparation Time: 10 minutes

Cooking Time: 15 minutes

Servings: 8

Ingredients:

- 2 eggs
- 2 cups almond flour
- 2 tbsp. coconut oil, spray
- 2 eggplants, peeled and cut thinly
- Salt and pepper

Directions:

1. Preheat your oven to 400°F.
2. Take a bowl and mix with salt and black pepper in it.
3. Take another bowl and beat eggs until frothy.
4. Dip the eggplant pieces into eggs.
5. Then coat them with a flour mixture.
6. Add another layer of flour and egg.
7. Then, take a baking sheet and grease with coconut oil on top.
8. Bake for about 15 minutes.
9. Serve and enjoy.

Nutrition:

- Calories: 212,
- Fat: 15.8 grams,
- Carbohydrates: 12.1 grams,
- Protein: 8.6 grams

5. Parmesan Crisps

Preparation Time: 5 minutes

Cooking Time: 25 minutes

Servings: 8

Ingredients:

- 1 tsp. butter
- 8 oz. parmesan cheese, full fat and shredded

Directions:

1. Preheat your oven to 400°F.
2. Put parchment paper on a baking sheet and grease with butter.
3. Spoon parmesan into 8 mounds, spreading them apart evenly.
4. Flatten them.
5. Bake for 5 minutes until browned.
6. Let them cool.
7. Serve and enjoy.

Nutrition:

- Calories: 133,
- Fat: 11 grams,
- Carbohydrates: 1gram,
- Protein: 11 grams

6. Low-Carb Brownies

Preparation Time: 10 minutes

Cooking Time: 20 minutes

Servings: 16

Ingredients:

- 7 tbsp. coconut oil, melted
- 6 tbsp. plant-based sweetener
- 1 large egg
- 2 eggs yolk
- ½ tsp. mint extract
- 5 oz. sugar-free dark chocolate
- ¼ cup plant-based chocolate protein powder
- 1 tsp. baking soda
- ¼ tsp. sea salt
- 2 tbsp. vanilla almond milk, unsweetened

Directions:

1. Start by preheating the oven to 350°F and then take an 8x8 inch pan and line it with parchment paper, being sure to leave some extra sticking up to use later to help you get them out of the pan after they are cooked.

2. Into a medium-sized vessel, use a hand mixer, and blend 5 tablespoons of the coconut oil (save the rest for later), as well as the egg, Erythritol, egg yolks, and the mint extract all together for 1 minute. After this minute, the mixture will become a lighter yellow hue.

3. Take 4 ounces of the chocolate and put it in a (microwave-safe) bowl, as well as with the other 2 tablespoons of melted coconut oil.

4. Cook this chocolate and oil mixture on half power, at 30-second intervals, being sure to stir at each interval, just until the chocolate becomes melted and smooth

5. While the egg mixture is being beaten, add the melted chocolate mixture into the egg mixture until this becomes thick and homogenous.

6. Add in your protein powder of choice, salt, baking soda, and stir until homogenous. Then, vigorously whisk your almond milk in until the batter becomes a bit smoother.

7. Finely chop the rest of your chocolate and stir these bits of chocolate into the batter you have made.

8. Spread the batter evenly into the pan you have prepared, and bake this until the edges of the batter just begin to become darker, and the center of the batter rises a little bit. You can also tell by sliding a toothpick into the middle, and when it comes out clean, it is ready. This will take approximately 20 to 21 minutes. Be sure that you do NOT over-bake them!

9. Let them cool in the pan they cooked in for about 20 minutes. Then, carefully use the excess paper handles to take the brownies out of the pan and put them onto a wire cooling rack.

10. Make sure that they cool completely, and when they do, cut them, and they are ready to eat!

Nutrition:

- Calories 107
- Fats 10g
- Carbohydrates 5.7g
- Protein 2.5g

7. Roasted Broccoli

Preparation Time: 5 minutes

Cooking Time: 20 minutes

Servings: 4

Ingredients:

- 4 cups broccoli florets
- 1 tbsp. olive oil
- Salt and pepper to taste

Directions:

1. Preheat your oven to 400°F.
2. Add broccoli in a zip bag alongside oil and shake until coated.
3. Add seasoning and shake again.
4. Spread broccoli out on the baking sheet, bake for 20 minutes.
5. Let it cool and serve.

Nutrition:

- Calories: 62,
- Fat: 4 grams,
- Carbohydrates: 4 grams,
- Protein: 4 grams

8. Almond Flour Muffins

Preparation Time: 15 minutes

Cooking Time: 30 minutes

Servings: 8

Ingredients:

- 1/3 cup of pumpkin puree
- 3 eggs
- 2 tbsp. agave nectar
- 2 tbsp. coconut oil
- 1 tsp. vanilla extract
- 1 tsp. white vinegar
- 1 cup chopped fruits
- 1 tsp. baking soda
- ½ tsp. salt

Directions:

1. Preheat the oven to 350°F.
2. Line the muffin tin with paper liners.
3. In the first mixing bowl, whisk the almond flour, salt, and baking soda.

4. In the second mixing bowl, whisk the pumpkin puree, eggs, coconut oil, agave nectar, vanilla extract, and vinegar.
5. Now add this puree mix of the second bowl to the first bowl and blend everything well.
6. Add the chopped fruits to the blend.
7. Pour the mixture into the muffin cups in your pan.
8. Bake for 15-20 minutes. Ensure that the contents have been set in the center, and a golden-brown lining has started to appear at the edges.
9. Transfer the muffins to a cooling rack and let them cool completely.

Nutrition:

- Calories: 75,
- Carbs: 4 grams,
- Fat: 6 grams,
- Protein: 0 gram

Chapter 11. Poultry and Meat

9. Barbeque Pork Ribs

Preparation Time: 10 minutes

Cooking Time: 60 minutes

Servings: 4

Ingredients:

- 2-2 ½ lb. pork spareribs or baby back ribs
- 1 tsp. liquid smoke (optional)
- ½ cup low carb barbecue sauce + extra to serve
- 2 tbsp. Dijon mustard
- ½ cup spice rub

Directions:

1. Place a sheet of aluminum foil on a rimmed baking sheet. Place a wire rack over it.
2. Place the ribs on the rack with the meat side facing up. Do not overlap.
3. Add mustard and liquid smoke into a bowl and stir. Brush this mixture all over the ribs.
4. Sprinkle dry rub over the ribs and press lightly so that the rub sticks onto the ribs.

5. Place in a preheated oven with a broiler setting. Broil until the ribs are brown.

6. Place a rack in the center of the oven. Shift the ribs onto this rack.

7. Bake in a preheated oven at 300°F for 2-3 hours if using spareribs or for 1 ½ -2 hours if using baby back ribs.

8. Cover the ribs with foil when the meat is half cooked.

9. Baste with barbecue sauce during the last 30 minutes of cooking. Cover and continue baking.

10. To check if the meat is cooked, insert a knife in the thickest part of the meat. If it pierces easily, the meat is cooked else cook it for some more time.

11. When done, let the meat sit for 10 minutes. Do not remove the foil during this time.

12. Uncover and place on your cutting board. When cool enough to handle, separate the ribs by cutting in between the bones.

13. Serve with extra barbecue sauce.

Nutrition:

- Calories 200,
- Fat 8g,
- Fiber 2g,
- Carbs 8g,
- Protein 6g

10. Paprika Lamb Chops

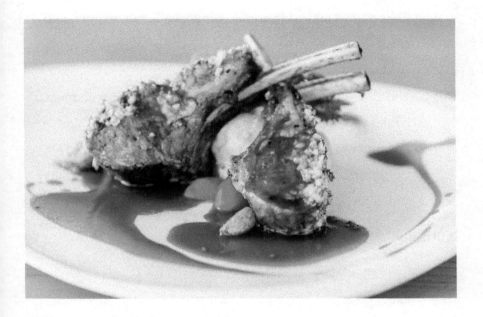

Preparation Time: 10 minutes

Cooking Time: 15 minutes

Servings: 4

Ingredients:

- 2 lamb racks, cut into chops
- Salt and pepper to taste
- 3 tbsp. paprika
- ¾ cup cumin powder
- 1 tsp. chili powder

Directions:

1. Take a bowl and add paprika, cumin, chili, salt, pepper, and stir.
2. Add lamb chops and rub the mixture.
3. Heat grill over medium-temperature and add lamb chops, cook for 5 minutes.
4. Flip and cook for 5 minutes more, flip again.
5. Cook for 2 minutes, flip and cook for 2 minutes more. Serve and enjoy.

Nutrition:

*   Calories: 200,
*   Fat: 5 grams,
*   Carbohydrates: 4 grams,
*   Protein: 8 grams

11. Delicious Turkey Wrap

Preparation Time: 10 minutes

Cooking Time: 10 minutes

Servings: 6

Ingredients:

- 1 and a ¼ lb. of ground turkey, lean
- 4 green onions, minced
- 1 tbsp. of olive oil
- 1 garlic clove, minced
- 2 tsp. of chili paste
- 8oz. water chestnut, diced
- 3 tbsp. of hoisin sauce
- 2 tbsp. of coconut amino
- 1 tbsp. of rice vinegar
- 12 butter lettuce leaves
- 1/8 tsp. of salt

Directions:

1. Take a pan and place it over medium heat, add turkey and garlic to the pan.
2. Heat for 6 minutes until cooked.
3. Take a bowl and transfer turkey to the bowl.

4. Add onions and water chestnuts.

5. Stir in hoisin sauce, coconut amino, vinegar, and chili paste.

6. Toss well and transfer the mix to lettuce leaves. Serve and enjoy.

Nutrition:

- Calories: 162,
- Fat: 4 grams,
- Carbohydrates: 7 grams,
- Protein: 23 grams

12. Bacon and Chicken Garlic Wrap

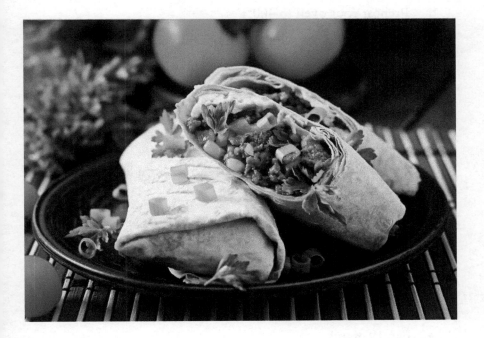

Preparation Time: 15 minutes

Cooking Time: 10 minutes

Servings: 4

Ingredients:

- 1 chicken fillet, cut into small cubes
- 8-9 thin slices bacon, cut to fit cubes
- 6 garlic cloves, minced

Directions:

1. Preheat your oven to 400°F.
2. Line a baking tray with aluminum foil.
3. Add minced garlic to a bowl and rub each chicken piece with it.
4. Wrap bacon piece around each garlic chicken bite.
5. Secure with a toothpick.
6. Transfer bites to the baking sheet, keeping a little bit of space between them.
7. Bake for about 15-20 minutes until crispy. Serve and enjoy.

Nutrition:

- Calories: 260,
- Fat: 19 grams,
- Carbohydrates: 5 grams,
- Protein: 22 grams

13. Lamb Curry

Preparation Time: 10 minutes

Cooking Time: 4 hours

Servings: 6

Ingredients:

- 2 tbsp. grated fresh ginger
- 2 cloves, peeled and minced garlic
- 2 tsp. cardamom
- 1 peeled and chopped onion
- 6 cloves
- 1 lb. Lamb meat, cubed
- 2 tsp. cumin powder
- 1 tsp. garam masala
- ½ tsp. chili powder
- 1 tsp. turmeric
- 2 tsp. coriander
- 1 lb. spinach
- Canned – 14 oz. canned

Directions:

1. In a slow cooker, mix lamb with tomatoes, spinach, ginger, garlic, onion, cardamom, cloves, cumin, garam masala, chili, turmeric, and coriander.
2. Stir well. Cover and cook on high for 4 hours.
3. Uncover the slow cooker, stir the chili, divide into bowls, and serve.

Nutrition:

- Calories 181,
- Fat 9g,
- Fiber 5g,
- Carbs 8g,
- Protein 14g

14. Turmeric Rack of Lamb

Preparation Time: 15 minutes

Cooking Time: 16 minutes

Servings: 4

Ingredients:

- 13 oz. rack of lamb

- 1 tbsp. of ground turmeric

- ½ tsp. of chili flakes

- 3 tbsp. of olive oil

- 1 tbsp. of balsamic vinegar

- 1 tsp. of salt

- ½ tsp. of peppercorns

- ¾ cup of water

Directions:

1. In the shallow bowl, mix up together ground turmeric, chili flakes, olive oil, balsamic vinegar, salt, and peppercorns.
2. Brush the rack of lamb with the oily mixture generously.

3. After this, preheat the grill to 380°F.

4. Place the rack of lamb in the grill and cook it for 8 minutes from each side.

5. The cooked rack of lamb should have a light crunchy crust.

Nutrition:

- Calories 252

- Fat 18.8,

- Fiber 0.4,

- Carbs 1.3,

- Protein 18.9

15. Pork Carnitas

Preparation Time: 10 minutes

Cooking Time: 50 minutes

Servings:

Ingredients:

- Pepper
- ¼ tsp. salt
- ½ tbsp. dark molasses
- ½ tbsp. orange juice
- 1 tbsp. brown sugar
- 1 minced garlic clove
- ½ lb. pork tenderloin

Directions:

1. Rinse off the pork tenderloin and blot it down with some paper towels. Slice thinly and then set it aside.
2. Place a skillet on a flame or burner set to high, and then heat it up for about a minute. Once the skillet is hot, add the pork tenderloin. Cook these for about 4 minutes until the pork is tender and cooked throughout.
3. Drain out the oil before stirring in the pepper, salt, molasses, orange juice, and brown sugar.

4. Stir this around and simmer until your sauce is thick. Turn off the heat and let it stand for a few minutes to thicken before serving.

Nutrition:

- Calories 294,
- Fat 12g,
- Fiber 2g,
- Carbs 8g,
- Protein 45g

Chapter 12. Salad and Soups

16. Shrimp Salad

Preparation Time: 15 minutes

Cooking Time: 0 minutes

Servings: 8

Ingredients:

- 1/3 English cucumber, diced
- ¾ cup plain yogurt
- 1 lb. shrimp, cooked & chopped
- 1 tbsp. Dijon mustard
- 1 tsp. garlic powder
- 2 tbsp. mayo
- 3 med. stalks celery, diced
- Sea salt & pepper, to taste

Directions:

1. Mix thoroughly all ingredients in a bowl.
2. Cover and put in the fridge for 15 minutes before serving.
3. Serve chilled!

Nutrition:

- Calories 112
- Carbohydrates 4g
- Fat 5g
- Protein 14g

17. Broccoli Salad

Preparation Time: 20 minutes

Cooking Time: 5 minutes

Servings: 6

Ingredients:

- ½ cup dried cranberries, unsweetened
- ½ cup pecans, chopped
- ½ cup sunflower seeds
- 1 ½ tbsp. onion powder
- 1 cup plain yogurt
- 1 lb. broccoli, chopped
- 1 small bell pepper, diced
- 1 tbsp. apple cider vinegar
- Red pepper flakes, to taste
- Sea salt & pepper, to taste

Directions:

1. In a medium bowl, thoroughly mix all ingredients.
2. Cover and refrigerate for 15 minutes before serving.
3. Serve chilled!

Nutrition:

- Calories 234
- Carbohydrates 20g
- Fats 13g
- Protein 9g

18. Southwest Chicken Salad

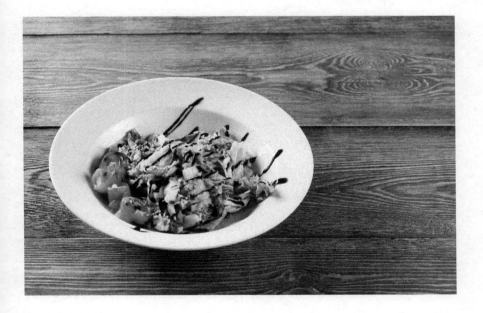

Preparation Time: 15 minutes

Cooking Time: 15 minutes

Servings: 8

Ingredients:

- ¼ cup extra virgin olive oil
- ¼ cup red onion, finely chopped
- 1 cup corn, drained
- 1 can low-sodium black beans, rinsed & drained
- 1 jalapeño, seeded & minced

- 1 tsp. chili powder

- 1 tsp. cumin

- 1 tsp. garlic powder

- 1 tsp. onion powder

- 2 bell peppers, diced

- 2 lg. limes, juiced

- 2 lb. chicken thighs, cooked and diced

- 2 tbsp. cilantro, finely chopped

- 3 cup quinoa, cooked

- Sea salt & black pepper, to taste

Directions:

1. In a small bowl, mix chili powder, lime juice, onion powder, garlic powder, cumin, and cilantro. Mix thoroughly and set aside.

2. In a large mixing bowl, combine all other ingredients and toss until thoroughly combined.

3. Drizzle seasoning mixture over the salad and toss to coat completely.

4. Cover and refrigerate for 30 minutes before serving.

19. Tuna Salad

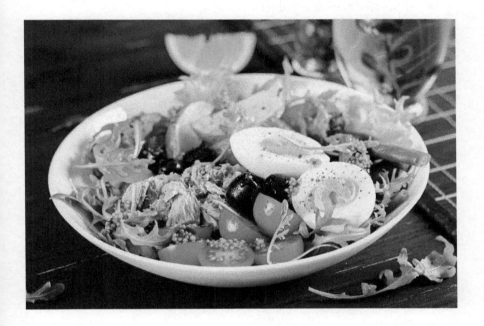

Preparation Time: 15 minutes

Cooking Time: 0 minutes

Servings: 10

Ingredients:

- ¼ cup mayonnaise
- ¼ cup red onion, finely diced
- ¾ cup plain yogurt
- 1 clove garlic, minced
- 1 lg. stalk celery, diced

- 1 tbsp. lemon juice

- 2 small dill pickles, diced

- 24 oz. tuna packed in water, drained

- Sea salt & pepper, to taste

Directions:

1. In a medium bowl, thoroughly mix all ingredients.

2. Chill in the fridge for 12 minutes while covered before serving.

3. Serve chilled!

Nutrition:

- Calories 152

- Carbohydrates 2g

- Fats 8g

- Protein 18g

20. Greek Quinoa Salad

Preparation Time: 10 minutes

Cooking Time: 15 minutes

Servings: 6

Ingredients:

- ¼ cup red onion, finely chopped
- ½ cup feta cheese crumbles
- ½ cup parsley, finely chopped
- ½ English cucumber, chopped
- 1 cup quinoa, cooked and cooled
- 1 lemon, juiced
- 1 large bell pepper, chopped
- 1 medium tomato, diced
- 1 tbsp. cumin
- 2 tbsp. extra virgin olive oil
- 20 Kalamata olives pitted and halved
- Sea salt & pepper, to taste

Directions:

1. In a medium bowl, thoroughly mix all ingredients.
2. Cover and chill in the fridge for 15 minutes before serving.

Nutrition:

- Calories 344
- Carbohydrates 28g
- Fat 23g
- Protein 8g

21. Asparagus and Green Peas Salad:

Preparation Time: 10 minutes

Cooking Time: 30 minutes

Servings: 2

Ingredients:

- 1 cup green peas
- 1 carrot, chopped
- 1 lb. asparagus trimmed
- 1 bunch frisee
- 1 red onion, chopped
- 1 rib celery, chopped
- 1 tbsp. flaxseed oil
- ½ tbsp. Dijon mustard
- 2 tbsp. balsamic vinegar
- 1 tbsp. extra-virgin olive oil
- ½ cup goat cheese, crumbled

Directions:

1. Preheat the oven to 4500°F.
2. Pour 3 cups of water into a large saucepan and bring to a boil. Add in onion lentils, carrots, and celery. Reduce heat and

allow to simmer for 15 minutes or until the lentils are tender. Drain. Set aside.

3. Meanwhile, layer asparagus on a baking sheet. Tilt sheet to roll asparagus to coat with cooking spray. Roast for 15 minutes.

4. In another bowl, put together mustard and balsamic vinegar. Whisk in flaxseed oil and olive oil. Mix well. Drizzle in lentil mixture. Toss until well coated.

5. To serve, arrange fries on plates. Put a lentil mixture and sprinkle goat cheese.

Nutrition:

- Calories 156,
- Fat 8g,
- Fiber 2g,
- Carbs 8g,
- Protein 56g

22. Quick and Easy Squash Soup:

Preparation Time: 5 minutes

Cooking Time: 15 minutes

Servings: 1

Ingredients:

- 1tbsp. of olive oil
- 1 cup of chopped onions
- 1 cup of chopped squash
- 2 cups of chicken broth
- ½ tsp. of nutmeg
- ½ tsp. of salt
- 1 tsp. of pepper

Directions:

1. Deposit your 1 tablespoon of olive oil into a large saucepan, before adding your 1 cup of chopped onions, your 1 cup of chopped squash, your 2 cups of chicken broth, your ½ teaspoon of nutmeg, your ¼ teaspoon of salt, and your 1 teaspoon of pepper.
2. Stir everything together well and cook for 15 minutes under high heat.
3. Serve when ready!

Nutrition:

- Calories 108,
- Fat 8g,
- Fiber 2g,
- Carbs 8g,
- Protein 7g

Chapter 13. Fish and Seafood

23.Light Fish Stew

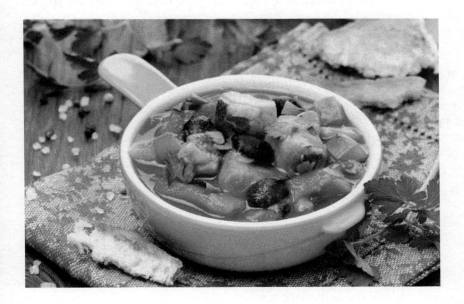

Preparation Time: 10 minutes

Cooking Time: 25 minutes

Servings: 4

Ingredients:

- 4 slices of brown bread cut into cubes. Make sure the bread is old, e.g., stale

- 2 tbsp. olive oil

- 1 onion, chopped very finely

- 2 cloves of garlic, crushed and chopped

- 1 tsp. chili flakes, dried

- 1 x 400g can of tomatoes, chopped

- 4 fillets of white fish, e.g., pollock or cod. You can use frozen here also

- 1 x 400g can have drained butter beans

- A little parsley, chopped

Directions:

1. Preheat your oven to 200°C

2. Take a large baking sheet and add a little of the oil over the top

3. Arrange the bread onto the baking sheet and place it in the oven for 10 minutes

4. Once cooked, place it to one side

5. Take a large casserole dish (flameproof) and add the remaining oil, heat over a medium heat

6. Add the onions and allow to cook for around 10 minutes

7. Add the chili flakes and the garlic and combine, cooking for a further minute

8. Add the tomatoes and combine

9. Now add the fish and place a lid over the top of the dish

10. Simmer for 10 minutes, and then take the lid off

11. Add the butter beans and season with salt and pepper

12. Continue cooking until the fish is cooked and everything is soft

13. Add the bread pieces and serve with a little chopped parsley

Nutrition:

- Calories 210,
- Fat 8g,
- Fiber 2g,
- Carbs 8g,
- Protein 7g

24. Lemon Baked Salmon

Preparation	Cooking Time:	Servings:	2
Time: 5 minutes	20 minutes		

Ingredients:

- 12 oz. filets of salmon
- 2 lemons, sliced thinly
- 2 tbsp. Olive oil
- Salt and black pepper, to taste
- 3 sprigs thyme

Directions:

1. Preheat the oven to 350°F.
2. Place half the sliced lemons on the bottom of a baking dish.
3. Place the fillets over the lemons and cover with the remaining lemon slices and thyme.
4. Drizzle olive oil over the dish and cook for 20 minutes.
5. Season with salt and pepper.

Nutrition:

- Calories 571,
- Fat 44g,
- Fiber 2g,
- Carbs 2g,
- Protein 42g

25. Easy Blackened Shrimp

Preparation Time: 10 minutes

Cooking Time: 6 minutes

Servings: 2

Ingredients:

- ½ lb. shrimp, peeled and deveined
- 2 tbsp. blackened seasoning
- 1 tsp. olive oil
- Juice of 1 lemon

Directions:

1. Toss all ingredients (except oil) together until shrimp are well coated.
2. In a non-stick skillet, heat the oil to medium-high heat.
3. Add shrimp and cook 2-3 minutes per side.
4. Serve immediately.

Nutrition:

- Calories 152,
- Fat 4g,
- Fiber 1g,
- Carbs 8g,
- Protein 24g

26. Grilled Shrimp Easy Seasoning

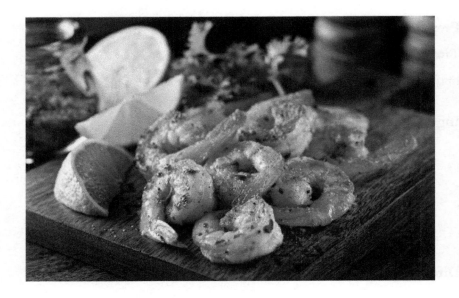

Preparation Time: 5 minutes

Cooking Time: 5 minutes

Servings: 4

Ingredients:

Shrimp Seasoning:

- 1 tsp. garlic powder
- 1 tsp. kosher salt
- 1 tsp. Italian seasoning
- ¼ tsp. cayenne pepper

Grilling:

- 2 tbsp. olive oil
- 1 tbsp. lemon juice
- 1 lb. jumbo shrimp, peeled, deveined
- Ghee for the grill

Directions:

1. Preheat the grill pan to high.
2. In a mixing bowl, stir together the seasoning ingredients.
3. Drizzle in the lemon juice and olive oil and stir.
4. Add the shrimp and toss to coat.
5. Brush the grill pan with ghee.
6. Grill the shrimp until pink, about 2-3 minutes per side.
7. Serve immediately.

Nutrition:

- Calories 101,
- Fat 3g,
- Fiber 1g,
- Carbs 1g,
- Protein 28g

27. The Best Garlic Cilantro Salmon

Preparation Time: 10 minutes	Cooking Time: 15 minutes	Servings: 4

Ingredients:

- 1 lb. salmon filet
- 1 tbsp. butter
- 1 lemon
- ¼ cup fresh cilantro leaves, chopped
- 4 cloves garlic, minced
- ½ tsp. kosher salt
- ½ tsp. freshly cracked black pepper

Directions:

1. Preheat oven to 400°F.
2. On a foil-lined baking sheet, place salmon skin side down.
3. Squeeze lemon over the salmon.
4. Season salmon with cilantro and garlic, pepper and salt.
5. Slice butter thinly and place pieces evenly over the salmon.
6. Bake for about 7 minutes, depending on thickness.
7. Turn the oven to broil and cook for 5-7 minutes, until the top is crispy.
8. Remove salmon from the oven and serve immediately.

Nutrition:

- Calories 140,
- Fat 4g,
- Fiber 2g,
- Carbs 3g,
- Protein 20g

Conclusion

In anything new that we attempt, quite possibly, we may stumble. Fasting or following another eating routine plan is the same. The target ought not to be on the way that you stumbled but on how you choose to return and approach it once more. You need not quit if you have a day or two where you didn't achieve your full fast. You simply need to re-evaluate your plan and approach it differently.

Perhaps your fasting period was excessively long for your first attempt. Possibly you're fasting and eating windows didn't coordinate with your sleep/ wake cycle as well as they could have. Any of these variables can be changed following what better suits you. You have several options to adapt according to your lifestyle. With the human body, there will never be a right or a wrong method to approach.

It is always a good idea to talk with a certified medical care expert before rolling out dietary improvements, regardless of whether you are simply changing the circumstance of when you eat foods. They can assist you in deciding whether intermittent fasting would be valuable for you. This is particularly significant for longer-term diets in which vitamin and mineral exhaustion may happen.

Understand that our bodies are amazingly smart. If the food is restricted at one meal, the body can build a hunger, and the measure of Calories devoured at the following meal, and even slow down digestion to coordinate with calorie utilization. Intermittent fasting has numerous potential medical advantages, yet it ought not to be expected that whenever followed carefully, it is ensured to create gigantic weight reduction and forestall the turn of events or movement of illness. It is a valuable tool; however, numerous instruments may be implemented to help in accomplishing and keeping up the ideal.

This book is a journey toward a healthy lifestyle. It has shown you how numerous factors are included concerning wellbeing and health. It is intended to inform you of plenty of alternatives that are accessible to you. Remember the numerous options that were spread out for you, including diet alternatives and explicit food sources that can actuate autophagy in the mind.

It is your work now to choose which of these food sources or improvements to remember for your life and to rehearse such experimentation, noticing which ones cause you to feel incredible and which ones you like to do without. With all of this data, you can choose which ways fit best with your particular way of life and your inclinations. As you take all this data forward with you, it might appear overpowering to start applying this into your own life. Keep in mind, life is a cycle, and you don't have to expect flawlessness from yourself. By finding a way to pursue this book, you are already transforming your life.

I hope that this book will give you all you need to know. There are numerous offers of delivery regarding this matter on the lookout, so thanks again for buying this book.

Lightning Source UK Ltd.
Milton Keynes UK
UKHW020848180521
383917UK00001B/109